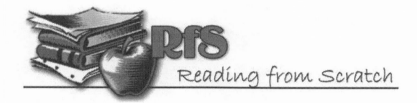

Reading from Scratch

Wiping Out Dyslexia

with

Enhanced Lateralization

Musings from My Forty Years of Wiping

by

Dorothy van den Honert

authorHOUSE®

AuthorHouse™
1663 Liberty Drive
Bloomington, IN 47403
www.authorhouse.com
Phone: 1-800-839-8640

Published by AuthorHouse   03/23/2012

ISBN: 978-1-4685-2810-7 (sc)
ISBN: 978-1-4685-2812-1 (hc)
ISBN: 978-1-4685-2811-4 (e)

Library of Congress Control Number: 2011962504

Dedicated

To

Dr. Michael Gazzaniga, whose phrase,

"-one final cognitive path"

was to dyslexia what penicillin is to pneumonia

RfS reading from scratch **THE DYSLEXIA SOLUTION**

Dorothy van den Honert 115 Mountain Drive Pittsfield, MA 01201 www.dyslexia.org

Tel: 413-442-2687

E-mail: info@dyslexia.org

PREFACE

A number of years ago there was a young couple living two houses up from us who were the kind of people who put their money where their mouths were. When they heard that children of half Korean, half GI parentage were outcasts in Korean society, they decided to adopt one. Five-year-old Tommy arrived at Kennedy Airport one April knowing "Mama," "Daddy," and "hungry," and that was about it. June and Dick could say "Mama," "Daddy," and "bathroom?" in Korean, and **that** was about it.

Tommy spent the summer making a mind-boggling adjustment to his new life. About the only things common to his two worlds were the blue sky and the general shape of human beings. Then in September, with a make-do supply of English under his little belt, he started in the first grade. He loved school. He loved the bright toys, the pictures in the books. He loved lunch and recess. But at the end of the year, his happy world nearly collapsed around his ears. The school decided that since he couldn't read, he would have to repeat first grade!

June couldn't bear to tell him. She was practically in tears as we talked about it over coffee one morning. It was so unfair. Tommy had worked like a Trojan. She knew that if he were kept back, he would feel that he had disgraced his new family, and he would be shamed horribly in the eyes of his friends. She just couldn't stand it.

Well, I couldn't stand it, either. Tommy was rather a favorite of mine. I had taught my own kids to read before they got to first grade, being no fan of the "look, say" method then in fashion, so I told June to talk the school into promoting him on the grounds that she would make sure he learned to read. Then I would teach him, myself.

And that's what we did. I got out the little book, *Reading with Phonics,* by Hay-Wingo, which I had used on my own five. Tommy came over after school for twenty minutes or so nearly every day. At the end of second grade, his teacher told June she was amazed at how well he was doing. Tommy was in the middle of his second grade class in reading! (June never let on that he was getting phonics straight up). What did I know about teaching reading? Not a thing. I was a math major in college. I just took the little book and went through it, word for word, until we got to the end.

Tommy was not dyslectic, so he was easy to teach. A dyslectic child needs more material, more exercises, and special techniques to learn to read. But if you can spare forty minutes three days a week during the school year, if you read all the directions in the *Reading from Scratch* material, follow them carefully and just go through it until you get to the end, you can do for a child what June and Dick did for Tommy: prevent him from growing up barred from a normal life in his own society. It is quite a gift.

CONTENTS

WIPING OUT DYSLEXIA

Musings from My Forty Years of Wiping

Right now about the only people who know how
many dyslectic kids there are in American schools are
statisticians. Teachers don't know. Parents don't know.
School Boards don't know. But if your bright little Alfie's
reading is a disaster that is messing up his life, somebody
besides statisticians better find out. The answer may
surprise you: dyslexia exists in fifteen to twenty percent
of the population! Any population.

Fortunately dyslexia can be wiped out. Not just
helped, modified, eased, or diluted. But if you say so to
a SPED teacher she will look at you funny. How I found
out about a genuine cure is a rather short story. Why so
few know about it and why so little is done about it is a
much longer and discouraging one.

Back in 1973 when the first of my five offspring
started to college, it was time for Mama to hit the road

and get a paid job. Teaching was an obvious choice because of the convenient hours, but with no education credits in my AB, I had to begin with subbing. It was fun until one afternoon during an eighth grade English class, a bunch of obstreperous boys in the back of the room began cutting up and making my life miserable. The ring-leader was a six footer with a shock of blond hair. Extremely irritated at the nerve of some 14 year old twit, I marched down the aisle to his desk, grabbed him by the hair, dragged him to the front of the room and shoved him out the door!

Well, that calmed the rest of the bad boys in a hurry. Later that afternoon there came a knock on the door of the art room where I was working. It was my blondie. Looking down at his feet, he said that Mr. Hickey (Vice Principal) had told him to apologize to me and he better make it sound genuine because if he didn't he wouldn't be walking across the stage with his class at graduation! Of course I swallowed a giggle, assured him that I wouldn't dream of spoiling his graduation, but added that it was on one condition: the next time he had a sub, he was to behave at least once! After that whenever he saw me, it was, "Good morning, Mrs. van den Honert," doors opened magically and we became friends.

A few months later in 1969, a regular teaching position opened up that nobody wanted. It was a class of six dyslexic boys who were climbing the walls with their frantic teacher right after them. Apparently I had gotten the reputation of being somebody who didn't take nothin' off nobody, because I was offered the job! Did I want it? Of course. The job was teaching them to read. Could I teach reading? Of course. I had taught my five little bookworms to read. These were dyslectic. Did I know anything about dyslexia? Never heard of it. But nobody else wanted the boys, so I got 'em. And that's how I backed into dyslexia, clueless.

I quickly discovered that dyslexia is no joke. It is bad enough in childhood, when bright children who just can't seem to read have to endure undeserved punishment from adults, teasing and rejection from friends, report cards bristling with accusatory F's, and generally lacerated egos. Even today the average dyslectic child spends his early life in schoolrooms where the teacher thinks he has an attitude or is stupid, doesn't try, cheats, won't sit still, loses his homework or can't concentrate. (By the way, it is unbelievably cruel to say that dyslectic kids don't try. They try until they are limp.) Nobody at any grade level wants his pals to think he is stupid, have the teacher make nasty remarks or laugh at his mistakes in class (yes, a lot of them do) or have a report card he wants to drop into the storm sewer after he gets off the bus. I once had a nice seventh grade boy who was Mr. Niceguy in my room and a menace in his English class. I'd have sworn he could throw a spitball before the teacher even knew she was going to call on him. I once asked him why he was so *bad* in her class. He answered patiently, "Mrs. van den Honert, would you rather be the kid who *can't* or the kid who *won't*? Some kids lash out and become behavior problems. Some just get depressed. Sometimes it gets worse. A teacher who has a squirmer may try to persuade the parent that the kid has ADD or ADHD (as if she knew the first thing about either one) and try to get the child on Ritalin or some other drug. You may be sure that Ritalin never taught a child to read.

Things don't improve much in adulthood. If I can't sing an aria, read Chinese, or tap dance, it doesn't depress me. My friends don't assume my ineptitude in these areas is due to lack of intelligence. But they do if I can't read. To an adult, dyslexia may mean going out to a restaurant and having to wait until his dinner partner orders so he an casually duplicate the order, only to get stuck with Fettucini Alfredo when he hates pasta. It can mean a lifetime of pretending and covering up, of hiding the lack of reading ability from employers, friends and family. For the dyslectic father of a dyslectic boy it can be worse, especially if Papa is in denial about a reading problem of his own. Daddy's male ego is threatened and often he takes it out in meanness to the boy or nasty teasing and hissy fits at poor report cards.

Years ago when Massachusetts realized that it had an awful lot of kids in school who for whatever reason couldn't learn at the average rate, they separated them into three categories: physically handicapped, mentally handicapped and dyslectic. Well you can bet your booties that the parents of the retarded kids didn't like that any, and they fussed until the Board of Education lumped everybody into something called "Children with Special Needs." The experts were surprised to find out that more than two thirds of these "children with special needs" were not retarded at all but bright kids with seriously substandard reading levels. If an intelligent seventh grader is reading at third grade level and he's not blind or deaf, whatever is holding up his reading and spelling capabilities is invisible.

And there is the the heart of the problem. Dyslexia is invisible. Having an invisibility cloak may be dandy for Harry Potter, but for the dyslectic student whose writing looks as though it originated in Outer Mongolia and who spells even worse than the average American, his annoyed teacher resorts to a laundry list of excuses that have, you understand, nothing to do with her teaching: the kid has an attitude, never listens, forgets everything, is distractible and cheats. He copies other students' work and puts the spelling words on the chair between his legs so he can use them for the test. For years

"Treatment" for these oddball kids was as oddball as the kids. It encompassed such interesting things as jumping on trampolines, taking megavitamins or motion sickness pills, looking through colored lenses, being in a resource room stuck with an "inclusion" model, and worst of all, of course, being pumped full of ritalin. To this day, I have still heard "experts" in the field maintain that a dyslectic child will never achieve grade-level reading! (Good manners prevent me from commenting on that one.)

I didn't know any of this my first day with the boys, but as I reached for some material the previous teacher had left me, at least I began to find out about lacerated egos in a hurry.

"Aw gee, do we have to read that stuff?" asked a lanky fourteen year old.

"Why no, Tommy. You don't have to read anything you don't like. What's the matter with this stuff?" I asked somewhat surprised.

"You know what it says in there?" he said, looking at it with distaste. "This—is—a—horse!" and he strung out the words with disgust.

I looked at the six pairs of eyes staring at me from around the table. Two of the boys had already spent a year in reform school when they were ten. Another had emotional problems from hydrocephalus. Two pairs of eyes belonged to the haunted faces of children who hadn't

6

"measured up" to educated parents' expectations. Three of these seventh graders were already taller than I was.

"This—is—a—horse?"

No.

"Well, I don't plan to bore you all to death, and I don't plan to bore myself to death either, so I guess we'll throw this out and get something better," I said cheerfully, and a sigh of relief went around the table.

Two days later during math class I got my second lesson in lacerated egos. In those days we operated sitting around a table in the corner of the school library since we didn't have a room of our own. I had distributed Cuisenaire rods to everybody, and each student had taken a piece of yellow paper from the pile in the center to do his calculations. Hearing the door of the library open, I glanced around and saw a ninth grade English class piling in. When I turned back, there were six innocent faces looking at me over yellow papers that were scattered all over the table. Nary a Cuisenaire rod was visible. For the next twenty minutes until the English class left, we sat around the scattered papers and blandly discussed the latest ball scores, the possibility of snow and the international situation. Finally the last of the ninth graders left. The yellow papers were neatly returned to the center of the table, the rods magically reappeared, and math class went on without a word from me.

Dismayed at the thought of having to give up Cuisenaire rods, I pointed out to the boys that the rods are not toys at all, but math tools, and that some very good schools use them all the way up to algebra. Patiently Tommy explained.

"Yeah, we know that, and you know that, but the other kids don't."

So I gave up the rods with a sigh until we could have private quarters and started looking for more suitable reading material. But all the reading programs were for elementary school, filled with stories in big print about puppies and kiddies. Grimly, I settled on the specifications of the material I wanted. It would be phonics, straight up, appear adult on quick inspection from a passing pal (no pictures, no print bigger than typing), and would use a vocabulary that would not insult a reasonably cool fourteen-year-old. (*Hubcap* is just as simple phonetically as *kitten.* "He flipped his lid," may not be Shakespeare, but it certainly beats, "Oh, see the red wagon!")

Obviously I wound up pounding out my own material and lived quite awhile on index cards and piles of loose blue ditto sheets. My program had an adult vocabulary from its first page of three letter words and was my contribution to healing lacerated egos. I had made it clear from the second day of class that I knew the boys were intelligent, but something odd was holding up their reading and I aimed to find out what it was.

That summer I took an intensive course in dyslexia which was no help. It told all about the symptoms, which I already knew, the need for phonics, which I had already begun and stated frankly that grade-level reading was probably out of the question in spite of years of individual help, which I didn't want to believe. So I skipped the courses and began to dig into a bit of history.

When the Russian spacecraft Sputnik blasted off in 1957 to become the first man-made object successfully put into orbit, it left science teaching in the schools of America red-faced. One disgruntled taxpayer couldn't resist the temptation to calculate the average time lag between discoveries in brain science and their application to education. He came up with a figure of about 50 years. In the case of dyslexia he was off by about another thirty. The gap between the discovery of dyslexia and an effective treatment for it was closer to 80 years. At least there was a good excuse for part of this gap because back 80 years ago it didn't really matter whether you could read well or not as long as you weren't going to go into one of the professions. The rest of mankind could make a nice living courtesy of the Industrial Revolution in factories and farms with minimum educational requirements.

Nobody blanched at the 90% high-school dropout rate of the early 1900's and illiteracy was not even noticed during the great depression because the whole world was in a pickle.

But the Second World War required more and more elaborate equipment for the military. The Technology Revolution supplanted the Industrial Revolution and the need for good reading to hold a job became painfully apparent. Educators responded with an educational disaster called "Whole Language" which produced a couple of generations of sloppy readers, conveniently camouflaging the dyslectic ones. Some misguided soul decided that it was more efficient if you read the whole word as a sort of picture instead of analyzing the phonetic construction. What he didn't know was that this put the process straight into the *right hemisphere where there is no grammar, no phonics, no sentence construction, no awareness of tenses, and no spelling. Where comprehension is slippery. "Skirt" is not "Shirt" "House" is not "horse," even though they have similar looks.* During the height of the "Whole Language" craze worldwide reading tests actually put the United States next to the bottom of the list with only Sri Lanka scoring worse!

With the predictable swing of the pendulum that characterizes educational theories, Whole Language mercifully disappeared. Phonics came back in fashion and miraculously American kids began to learn to read again with their left language areas. But the dyslectic ones didn't. Suddenly they stuck out of the crowd, invisible no longer and finally countable, often soaked in phonics—and still not reading.

But why? Nobody had a clue. These students were not slow. But you can't tell whether somebody is dyslexic just by looking at him. Nor, in those days could you peek into the inside of his head to see whether it was constructed normally. Hence the history of how science identified the real cause of dyslexia is a very boring story because for eighty or more years there was nothing to say.

Well, almost nothing.

To my surprise, I found that dyslexia had actually been identified by Samuel Orton as a separate phenomenon way back in 1925, but even eighty years later, almost nobody in the educational field had a clue as to what it was, never mind what to do about it. Orton was one of the first to realize that there were bright people with a strange reading problem that had nothing to do with intelligence, and he was right in that. But he was wrong in thinking that when someone with "strephosymbolia," as he called it, misread *was* for *saw* it was because the right hemisphere was doing "mirror reading" or reversing the letters. It was a good guess considering that the real cause was still invisible. Wrong or not, it stuck, and to this day people will tell you that dyslectics read words backwards.

Many years later another piece of the puzzle turned up that implicated a bridge of tissue in the middle of the brain called the corpus callosum. The job of the corpus callosum is to be a connecting link between the two hemispheres, sending what comes into side A over to side B and vice versa so that the whole brain knows what's going on. A psychiatrist in Boston University named Dr. William Condon had been experimenting with high-speed photography of athletes. As a side line, he began taking high-speed movies of dyslectic and autistic children and discovered one of the most important clues to the problem of dyslexia. It seems that dyslectic children are out of sync with themselves right down the midline of the body. When they blink, one eyelid starts down a few milliseconds before the other. When they smile, one corner of the mouth starts up the same number of milliseconds before the other. When they turn toward a click, one side begins to turn the same number of milliseconds before the other. It all happens so fast that it takes high-speed photography to catch it. But apparently one side of the brain is getting the primary signal and then some milliseconds later, a secondary, weaker one comes across that slow corpus callosum from the other side. Because the time delay is the same size for each activity—visual, auditory, or kinesthetic,—he concluded that a second signal must be coming across the CC late. The psychiatrist's theory was confirmed years later when some of the first brain scans showed that in the dyslectic brain, the CC was, indeed, a slow transmitter of information. And the clever Dr. Condon's estimate of the delay, somewhere between 100 and 200 milliseconds, turned out to match the fancier measurements from hi-tech scans!

For the next twenty years I combed the neurology journals for answers, but the flood of the new research in neurology was not directed at the plight of hapless dyslectics. Instead, hints about what might account for their reading problem came dribbling in in dribs and drabs of disconnected pieces of information, from every field you can think of except reading research. Like pieces of a jigsaw puzzle, one piece of information would turn out to fit another little piece if you happened to be looking for it. But virtually nobody gathered it all up and morphed it into effective teaching techniques because each specialist was looking for pieces of his own puzzle. For years isolated bits of technical information drifted in from:

1. the research using high speed photography on athletes (!)

2. anomalous double regressions and jerkiness in dyslectic eye motions
3. research on magno and parvo cells in the visual and auditory systems
4. realization of the plasticity of the brain
5. efforts to develop 3-D television
6. depression
7. ADD and ADHD
8. studies on stroke victims
9. a measurable timing delay of signal transfer across the corpus callosum

When scientists in one field didn't connect bits of their own information to the results from other people's fields they didn't recognize an underlying pattern that connected them all to dyslexia. The pattern turned out to be a sticky corpus callosum.

WHEN LEFT IS RIGHT

When I came across an article in Scientific American by Michael Gazzaniga, "The Split Brain in Man," I felt a prickle on the back of my neck. Apparently an epileptic seizure occurs when a neurological storm in one hemisphere crosses the bridge between the hemispheres and reaches the other side. In a few intractable cases Dr. Gazzaniga had resorted to surgically splitting the corpus callosum so that the two hemispheres were isolated from each other and transfer between them was impossible. It worked.

I didn't care about epilepsy, but what gave me the prickle was that with the two sides isolated, the doctors could find out what kinds of things each side was specialized for. And it seemed that the left hemisphere was specialized for the five things that my gang couldn't do: phonics, phonemic awareness, syntax, grammar, and letter sequencing. In a word, reading and spelling. Not long afterwards, in a lecture on dyslexia, Dr. Gazzaniga suggested that in dyslexia there was a lack of what he called, "one final cognitive path" for reading in the left hemisphere of the brain of the dyslectic reader. He felt that someone should find a way to isolate that left side and train it. He had been able to train his split-brained monkeys to use whichever side he chose.

Interesting. Splitting the brain is not an option for public school teachers, however tempting now and then. But the boys lucked out. I decided to see whether there would be a way I could just isolate lessons to the left hemisphere by distracting the right one to keep it out of the action.

About the same time, a research paper was published by a neurologist named Doreen Kimura who was interested in the importance of selective attention in learning. She put subjects into earphones with different words coming into the two ears simultaneously. On the first go around, they wrote what they heard in the right ear first and the left ear second. Then she switched it, having the left ear reporting first and the right ear second. She found that the ear that had the first report always had the most correct items. With this procedure each ear sends its signal directly to the opposite hemisphere and there it stays. No back-and-forth activity through a sticky corpus callosum. Apparently, *selective attention* then accounts for the difference in scores. Would it be possible by sending music to the right hemisphere and a phonics exercise to the left simultaneously, to stimulate and train the under-used left language area?

A bit more investigating turned up the most exciting information of all. Yes, when the two ears get qualitatively different inputs, like words and music, neither will ship its input to the other side. Bingo!

With two earplugs and two tape recorders, one recorder with a spelling exercise for one ear, the other recorder with some nice Mozart for the other ear, the boys were parked in the earplugs for fifteen minutes each day to write a list of words from dictation whose spelling rules I had (presumably) taught them. Signals are sent criss-cross in the brain, so the spelling words were delivered only to the right ear for transfer to the wimpy left hemisphere, while the nice Mozart went into the left ear for shipment across to the right hemisphere to keep it busy. In this way I hoped we could give private lessons to the left side.

Interestingly, when I was at a 2002 Rodin Dyslexia Conference in Munich, a Swedish teacher came up to me in a state of high excitement to talk about distracting one hemisphere while the other was given its phonics lesson. She had been doing something similar with astounding results and wanted to compare notes.

What she had done was to tape the evening news and use the talking heads' voices the next day for her right hemisphere distractor! The kids apparently thought it great fun to ignore the Important Person and she was getting improvement results that were on a par with mine. So perhaps just music isn't the only distractor that works, or even, if the Swedish lady is to be believed, the best one. Maybe the trick is that if the two sides hear different things, it is the *forced concentration* on the left hemisphere contents that makes the difference. Thank you, Dr. Kimura. In any case, you may be sure that I never wrote Dan Rather to tell him that a cohort of his listeners might be getting a surprising benefit from his wisdom if they made a real effort not to hear him.

When it came time to do something similar with vision, it looked more complicated. Each eye sends signals to both hemispheres. But you only have a language area on one side, so somebody has to ship its input across that corpus callosum. Apparently you can do it a couple of ways. You can ship only one direct signal across, which is what I did, or you can speed up the slow one so that both signals get there at the same time. Oddly enough, all you have to do to speed up the transfer is make the poky signal *brighter* than the on-time one. A psychiatrist in Mc Lean Hospital in Boston named Dr. Frederic Schiffer found that stimulating the left hemisphere of his depressed patients was extremely effective in treating depression. He developed some simple but ingenious glasses that enable a slightly brighter signal to go to the left hemisphere than to the right. Nearly all dyslectic people are somewhat depressed, usually from being considered damaged goods by their contemporaries.

And millions of kids are annually misdiagnosed with ADD or ADHD just because they can be twitchy and forgetful. So the calming and cheering effects are invaluable extras for dyslectic students. I put the boys in some of Dr. Schiffer's glasses to give the left hemisphere the brighter signal, and, indeed, it made reading easier for them.

Then I found a diagram of the visual system that showed something else that gave me the prickles. Each retina has two halves, one inside nearest the nose (the nasal retina) and the other outside toward the temples (the temporal retina, of course). What gave me the prickles is that *only the nasal retina ships what it sees directly to the opposite hemisphere without going through the CC.*

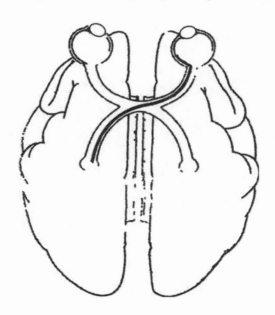

19

Maybe all I had to do was have the right nasal retina see a column of words while the left nasal retina couldn't see them! I took a piece of cardboard off a legal pad, scored the shorter side down about an inch in from the edge and bent it over and produced the original I-CARD! You can see from the picture that the bent strip blocks the left nasal retina but not the rest of the eye. So the left nasal retina never sees the words, while the right nasal retina dutifully ships them directly to the language area. (Figure 2). And that worked like gang-busters. A three year reading gain in one year of teaching became normal for the boys.

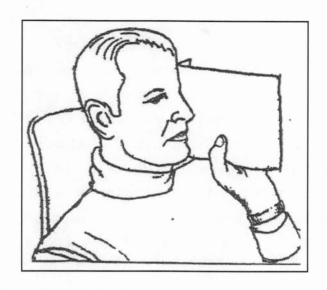

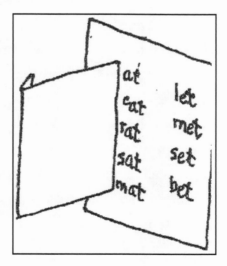

People who use the Reading from Scratch system often e-mail me to ask about what the peripheral vision is doing all this time. Here's my favorite way of explaining. A number of years ago, my mother was standing in line with an extra ticket for a Baltimore Symphony concert, and she found that the little old lady next to her only had a cheap SRO (standing room only) one. So my mother gave her the extra orchestra ticket and in they went. It was an interesting concert. The lady turned out to be the mother of the first trombonist. Every time he had a solo, his momma gave my mother a hefty poke with her elbow and said in a stage whisper, "DOT'S EDDY!" Of course Eddy's momma heard the rest of the orchestra while he was doing his bit, but she could never have told you what the violas were doing. She heard them, of course, but as Doreen Kimura pointed out, it's the selective attention that counts. The peripheral vision is like the rest of the orchestra. The brain takes in everything, but it is focused on only one thing at a time. Now you know why safety experts don't want you to be talking on your cell phone while you drive. The voice on the phone is Eddy's solo. The rest of the scene that is zipping past you at 40 mph is the orchestra.

And now for the next-to-last and probably the most important piece of our jigsaw puzzle. Neuroscientists who specialize in brain mapping have found that if two neurons sitting right next to each other from two different senses (vision and hearing in our case) are regularly stimulated by incoming signals *simultaneously*, chemical changes occur that make them connect with each other, effectively wiring them together. When that happens, they fire simultaneously, or, as one doctor put it, neurons that wire together fire together. But the timing is critical. Neurons out-of-sync fail to link, as he also so poetically put it. So when we use visual neurons that go to the left side directly so that they arrive *at the same time* as the auditory ones, over and over again, the two kinds of neurons begin to bond! Reading is, of course, both an auditory and a visual process. In dyslexia, the out-of-sync timing physically prevents wiring together the two senses necessary for reading. And it neatly accounts for the fact that the hallmark of dyslexia is the inability to match a sound with a symbol. Thank you, you poky CC.

Here is an interesting brain scan that shows the left hemisphere of two

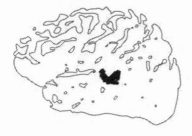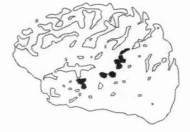

people. The left picture is from a normal reader, and the right one, a dyslectic reader. You can see how the neurons in the good reader cluster together and in the dyslectic reader are scattered all over.

So much for delayed visual input on one side. The other question is what it was about the CC that was making the auditory signals come across slowly. A number of researchers have found various areas where the CC is out of shape, and people have assumed that this may account for the slow interhemispheric timing. But that was guesswork. Finally, in 2002 a group of scientists in Bergen, Norway, took twenty dyslectic boys and twenty matched non-dyslectic boys, took pictures of their CC's and then traced the patterns onto paper so they could compare sizes and shapes directly. They found that 80% of the dyslectic boys could be easily identified because a central part of the CC, *the section that transmits auditory signals,* was too short! In fact, it was almost missing. Furthermore, proper development of that part of the brain accompanies a strong growth spurt in the later childhood years—just the time of literacy acquistion! Apparently that auditory area of the brain does not undergo the same growth pattern in dyslectics that it does in normal readers.

I hope that piece of information blew your mind, because it certainly blew mine when I read about it. How ironic that it took eighty years to find a bridge that can connect educators with scientists who are solving the problem. Talk about slow transmission! Eighty years for a few milliseconds' difference.

So there you have it. The source of dyslexia turns out to be a poky CC. (You might inform a principal who is giving you a hard time that dyslexia is the result of a dysfunctional corpus callosum that prevents synchronous interhemispheric transfer of visual and auditory signals, and let him figure it out.) In a nut shell, to get rid of dyslexia you must teach your pupil his phonics without using his corpus callosum.

Now here's a good question. If scientists know all this, how come teachers don't? Let me put it this way. Behold the title of the article from which I got the pictures you just saw. "Abnormal Activation of Temperoparietal Language Areas During Phonetic Analysis in Children With Dyslexia." Got it? Do you think if you read it that you would immediately think to fold in the edge of a piece of cardboard and give one side Beethoven and the other a spelling exercise? On the other hand it is not the job of scientists to turn their findings into teaching techniques.

Sadly there is just as big a gap in attitude between teachers and scientists as there is in the transfer of information between the two groups. Scientists only write in professional jargon, so they never bother to write in plain English. No PhD candidate ever wrote a chatty thesis. Someone reading a piece of research is expected to understand all the professional terms and mathematical analyses that prove the thesis. They write for each other.

Teachers think that scientists are ivory tower types who don't have a clue as to what is going on in the real world and what it needs. Teachers don't have time to learn the vocabulary of neurology so they can translate jargon. They'll tell you that scientists should started communicating in English with the people who can make their research useful.

The truth is that they are both half right and half wrong. History is replete with examples of discoveries not applied for centuries—and not always for lack of communication between inventor and user. Our disgruntled taxpayer was onto something. It is called human nature. People who already "know" something don't want to believe anything that counteracts what they already "know." Usually the first negative reaction is that "it" won't work. When Alexander Graham Bell tried to sell his telephone patent to Western Union, they turned it down on the gounds that "its commercial value will be limited." Indeed, a top journal of the industry at the time, *"The Telegrapher"* claimed that the telephone had "no direct application!" Xerox was said to "have no future." The first modern day helicopter design was rejected by the U. S. Patent Office in 1904 on the grounds of

"inoperativeness of the device for any useful purpose."
But my very favorite example of the granddaddy of all
gaps between known facts and application of them is
this: those ancient Greek geometers not only knew the
earth was round, they had figured out how big it was!
They actually knew all this nearly 2300 years before
Columbus hopped onto his boat and set out to prove the
same thing. So maybe a mere 80-year gap in recognizing
the importance of a few milliseconds' delay in crossing
the brain is not the worst example in human history!

WHY RIGHT IS WRONG

So now we know that the left hemisphere must be used for good reading, but we haven't explained why the right side can't do the same thing. To understand why right-brains make such a mess of reading, it helps to understand the specialties of the right hemisphere in the normal individual. The kinds of errors that characterize dyslectic reading are as follows:

- Difficulty with sound-symbol matching
- Disregard of punctuation
- Omission or inappropriate insertion of functors and abstract words (ifs, ands, althoughs, the's etc.)
- Poor letter-sequencing in spelling and reading
- Confusion of "b" and "d"
- Confusion of similar looking words, such as <u>form</u> and <u>from</u>
- Miscalling words by substituting non-phonetic synonyms: <u>ripped</u> for <u>torn</u>, <u>large</u> for <u>big</u>

- Omitting or miscalling syntactical endings, such as -ed, or -s.

In addition to this list, a dyslectic person will have at least some of the following *non-reading* problems:

- Left-right confusion
- Difficulty remembering a group of unrelated facts such as the multiplication table
- Difficulty remembering ordered lists such as the months of the year or the days of the week
- Impaired auditory sequential memory (following directions or repeating a long sentence) in the presence of normal visual sequential memory
- Difficulty understanding grammar or syntax, contributing to poor comprehension
- Measurably slow inter-hemispheric transfer of incoming signals
- Abnormal distractibility, "twitchiness" and hyperactivity
- Visual problems association with *motor control* of the eyes: lack of smooth tracking and convergence, poor stereopsis at the midline, and excessive eye fatigue with watering during reading
- Deficit in tactile localization

To make sense of this variety of peculiarities, you need to know something about how the standard brain works and how dyslectic processing differs, so that his reading comes out wrong, he can't remember directions and his eyes water.

Normally the two hemispheres share the mental work load, each with its own specialty. It is interesting to note that these specialties are usually hard-wired at birth. Even newborn babies use the left side to sort out and eventually understand language sounds, and the right side to begin to interpret environmental sounds: squeaks, horns, doors slamming, and the like. The corpus callosum sits in the middle like a traffic cop at a busy intersection, assigning tasks to the appropriate side for processing, supplying the focus to keep them in place, and sending split-second signals from one side to the other so that each one operates in sync with the other.

In the great majority of people (but not quite all), the left hemisphere is best at processing information that arrives in strings, one bit after the other, like the sounds in language. When you say CAT, the first noise you make is /k/, the second is /ă/, and the last is /t/. The order in which you say them makes a difference. CAT is not ACT. Keeping strings of incoming information in the proper lineup is a specialty of the left side. (When you are writing, it also prevents you from going "owdn" in an elevator after going "pu". No, I didn't make that up.)

On the other hand when you say, "It's all right here," what you mean depends on the tone of voice and the placement of emphasis. Think of the things that one phrase can mean. Just for fun, say that phrase in such a way that you mean:

"Hey, the weather's lovely here on Cape Cod even if you're in the middle of a sandstorm out there in Kansas." (It's all right HERE.)

"Everything you need is right where you dumped it in the middle of the floor." (IT'S ALL RIGHT HERE.)

Sorting out such subtle distinctions and keeping track of the emotional content of speech are specialties of the right hemisphere. So both sides of the brain are necessary for comprehension, each doing its own thing.

When it comes to deciphering written words, the principle of specialization holds. When the left hemisphere looks at a word, it is programmed to recognize the sound that each letter represents, produce the correct sequence of noises and come up with the word. It is also programmed to be able to use syntax, grammar and punctuation to extract the meaning of a sentence. For instance, in a sentence like, "The cat was bitten by the dog," the left side knows who did the biting even though that information is buried in the syntax of the passive voice. It knows that

-ed means something happened in the past, and that -ing represents something going on continuously. It has great respect for punctuation, realizing that the simple use of a question mark can turn a person into a cannibal.

"What are we having for supper tonight, Mother?"

"What are we having for supper tonight? Mother?" (And how would you like her, baked, boiled or fried?)

Or change an entire book: "Call me Ishmael." or "Call me, Ishmael." (Ring me up, Ish.)

In short, the left hemisphere is good at phonics, sequencing, and the use of syntax, grammar and abstract symbols that determine meaning.

The right hemisphere, on the other hand, is programmed to do none of the above. Its specialization is quite different. It is not built in such a way that it can match a visual mark with a language sound. If you take a pencil and do something on paper with it, the right brain sees the result as a pattern. The pattern may look like this:

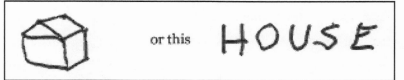

In either case, recognizing the meaning of the right hand pattern as a place where somebody lives, it might instruct your speech mechanism to say, "house."

Or maybe "home."

Or "residence," or maybe, "condo."

To the right brain, the lines in HOUSE form a line drawing that represents a concept: a place where somebody lives. The sketch does not represent a sound.

Similarly, the right brain can be taught that if it sees the line drawing, CAT, it is to think a small domesticated feline and if it sees RAT, it is to think an unwelcome brown rodent with a long skinny tail. But the right brain does not necessarily realize that those two "drawings" represent words that rhyme since it might just as well have been thinking kitty and rodent. It does not send a word that it sees through any sort of auditory loop to find out what the word sounds like.

Nor can the right side go the other way and turn sounds into letters. It cannot, for instance, spell nonsense words that it has never seen and whose spelling it has not memorized. If it can't read or spell "ex," "clu," or "sive," it will have trouble assembling them into <u>exclusive</u>. In fact, an excellent exercise for a pupil is to have him read lists of nonsense "words" like *norplat*, or *destab* that follow some spelling rule he has just learned. Drives 'em crazy! I love it.

To get a feeling for why it is so important to associate a sound with the word you are reading, try this trick. Look at the next page with the Hindi printing on it.

Note the word that is circled in the title. Now glance down the page and try to find the same word the next three times it appears in the text. You will discover that it takes an enormous amount of effort and eyestrain to find that pattern.

पष्ठ परिच्छेद

यहां (अंग्रेजी) बोली जाती है

धीरे-धीरे अंग्रेजी बोलने वाले लोगों ने उस सारे क्षेत्र पर अधिकार कर लिया जिसे आज संयुक्त राज्य कहा जाता है, और यही कारण है कि यहां रहने वाले हम लोग भी यह बात प्रायः भूल जाते हैं कि किन्हीं दूसरों जातियों ने इस देश की खोज करने तथा इसे बसाने के लिए बहुत बड़ा कार्य किया था।

यद्यपि सचाई यह है कि दो सौ वर्षों तक कोई यह न कह सकता था कि अंग्रेजी, स्पेनिश और फ्रेन्च में से कौन सी भाषा स्थायी रूप से अमेरिका के बोली जाएगी। हम पहले देख चुके हैं कि जब कोलम्बस ने अपनी यात्रा की, तब और उसके सौ वर्ष बाद तक भी केवल स्पेन और फ्रांस—ये दो देश ही यूरोप में वस्तुतः विशेष शक्तिशाली थे। पुर्तगाल तथा हालैण्ड का भी महत्व इंग्लैण्ड से अधिक था। जर्मनी तथा इटली का तो तब अस्तित्व ही न था। और उन प्रदेशों में अनेक छोटे-छोटे रजवाड़े बिखरे हुए थे जिनमें से कई अपने आपको राज्य, कुछेक डची या रियासत, दूसरे प्रिंसिपैलिटी अर्थात् सामन्तशाही और कई रिपब्लिक अर्थात् गणराज्य कहते थे। सुदूरपूर्व में एक प्रदेश ऐसा था जिसके विषय में यूरोप के दूसरे देश कुछ न जानते थे। वह तब मस्कोवी कहलाता था और उसका शासक एक महान ड्यूक था। जिन दिनों कोलम्बस ने अपनी यात्रा की थी, लगभग उन्हीं दिनों उस महान ड्यूक ईवान तृतीय ने मंगोलियन जाति के उन तातार लोगों को वहां से खदेड़ दिया, जहां वे कई शताब्दियों से जमे हुए थे और तब उसने एक नई उपाधि धारण की। वह ग्रैण्ड ड्यूक न रहा और मस्कोवी का कैसर बन गया। मास्को में उसे जार कहा जाता था। उन दिनों इस बिल्कुल प्रारम्भिक दशा में था और उसे बड़ी शक्ति बनने में कई शताब्दियां लग गईं।

१३१

35

Now do the same thing with the Portuguese text. Look for several repetitions of the word **HABIA**, that is on line two. This time it was easy. Your eye just went zip down the page and picked them all out with no trouble. Why? Because even if you don't know Portuguese, you automatically assigned a sound to that word and your brain quickly picked up that sound.

Hace quinientos años, en el territorio que es ahora Estados Unidos, no había una sola ciudad ni siquiera una casa de ladrillos; ningún camino pavimentado ni una fábrica ni un solo terreno arado. Por supuesto, no había ferrocarriles, automóviles ni aeroplanos, porque esas cosas no habían sido inventadas; pero, en otras partes del mundo, había muchas ciudades, caminos y campos. Había canales surcados por lanchones y ríos con grandes navíos. Había talleres donde hombres hábiles hacían cosas útiles y bellas. Había libros y pinturas, ropas hermosas, caballos y carruajes magníficos... en una palabra, la mayor parte de las cosas que la gente necesitaba para vivir cómodamente.

Pero eso ocurría en el hemisferio oriental. Si tomas un globo terráqueo y trazas una línea desde el Polo Norte a lo largo de la mitad del océano Atlántico hasta el Polo Sur y luego subes por la mitad del Pacífico hasta volver al Polo Norte, la parte del globo que contiene a Europa, Asia y África es el hemisferio oriental, y allí vivía la gente que había descubierto o inventado la mayor parte de las cosas que usamos diariamente.

En nuestra mitad del mundo, que llamamos el hemisferio occidental, hace quinientos años

But wasn't that because the English letters are more familiar? Only partly. English letters make it easier, but if you were to take a page and rewrite it with every word jumbled so that none of them were pronounceable, then tried the same trick, you would find it almost as difficult as finding the Hindi word. And you would find that you were trying your best to assign some sort of sound to what you were looking for. Look at a page in the mirror and try it. Again you will see that you are constantly trying to find a sound to attach to the word you are looking for.

(Yes, I have seen that game where the first and last letters of each word in a sentence are correct but the middle is all mixed up. People are surprised to find that they can often figure out the sentence, and then are told that the letter order doesn't matter when you read as long as the first and last letters are correct. That is a lotta baloney. You could not do the puzzle if you didn't know the words well in the first place. You have some clue in the first and last letters, and if you are a Jumbles fan who can do a quick anagram on them, you can get the sense of the sentence and come up with it.) It is true that the right hemisphere can memorize the shapes of a very large number of words. Some have estimated its capacity to be the size of a fifth grade vocabulary. It is also good at using context clues. It can make inferences and can often sort out subtle semantic differences between words. But for the sheer act of getting writing onto a sheet of paper and off again correctly, it is quite inept.

In addition to being useless at phonics, the right hemisphere has no framework of grammar or syntax into which it can place its words so that they make sense. In the sentence about the dog biting the cat the poor right brain would have no idea who the nasty one was because either one could bite the other and it doesn't understand the passive voice. On the other hand, it would have no trouble with the sentence, "The chocolate was eaten by the boy," because it doesn't need syntax to figure this out.

The right brain's ignorance of syntax also makes it poor at understanding those little "functor" words that glue pictorial nouns and verbs into sentences. It can comprehend dog, eyeball, sunset and coat hanger well enough since they can be visualized. But what about only, through, very, until, from, but? And what about commas, periods, quotation marks, apostrophes and semicolons? They're all abstract carriers of meaning, which means they're just mud in the eye of the right brain.

Before you get the impression that the right hemisphere is a total washout, I must admit that in many ways it is actually a lot cleverer than the left hemisphere.

It can handle mind-boggling (so to speak) amounts of information at a time. When you open your eyes and look at yourself in the mirror in the morning, your right brain sees and recognizes you, your disheveled hair, your coated tongue, the shape of the mirror and whatever else is reflect in it—the whole scene—in one pop. A gigantic amount of information is processed almost instantaneously. The right brain is also an expert at spatial relations. People with particularly well-developed right brains often become architects, inventors, artists, surgeons and engineers.

Now what does all this hemisphere stuff have to do with dyslectic people? When they read, they operate on language as if their *right* brains were running the show. Here are the kinds of peculiar things they do:

1. They make "semantic" errors, mistaking a word for its synonym—house for "home," black for "dark," Mom for "Mother," and the like. Note that there is no phonetic correspondence between the word and its synonym.
2. They romp merrily over periods and other punctuation marks as if such details don't exist.
3. They omit or insert functors and endings without batting an eye over what it does to the meaning of the sentence.

4. They make "look-alike" errors: "from" for "form," "passionate" for "patience," "devoured" for "devoted," "the reading" instead of "they realize."
5. They display short-term verbal memory deficits that are often severe.
6. Their spelling can only be described, in many cases, as bizarre.
7. They show very poor understanding of parts of speech or such things as passive voice or indirect objects.

Look at the letter below that was written to me by a bright young man of about thirty-five who was about to begin his lessons. His IQ was 138. This piece of writing is so typical of dyslexia that I have saved it to use it in all my workshops. Note such errors as the misplaced comma in the heading and the misplaced apostrophe in "Ia'm" in the third line. He knows visually that something goes there, but has no syntactical basis for deciding where the little mark goes. Also note the P.S. The man does not talk like that. When he uses "what" for wait, "pervious" for previous, "apperiate" for appreciate, and "passionate" for patience, (I loved that one!) he is clearly not using an auditory loop to spell.

Oct/8/81

Dear, Ms. VanDerbonet

    In enclosed is check for my perirous testing. I a'm waiting from answer from Mass Rehab. ony funding for contiueing classes. Sorry that it has taking so long for me to Asend out my pay- ment, Thank you for your passionate,

            Sincerely

P.s. probably you could give Mass Rehab to hurry with answer, I would appreate it. I can't what to start.

41

Now we must consider another list, this time of *non-reading* problems that also turn up regularly in healthy dyslectics. Much of the second list can be included in inappropriate right-hemisphere processing, too. In arithmetic, for instance, sequencing is critical. 13 is not 31; you must not subtract upside down, and the order of operations is crucial in things like long division. As to the infamous multiplication table, it is, to the right hemisphere, merely a jumble of disconnected abstractions. In addition to the language handling and math problems, remember the following oddities:

- Errors in Tactile Localization
- Abnormal distractibility, "twitchiness" and hyperactivity
- Problems with fine motor control, especially in handwriting
- Visual problems associated with *motor control* of the eyes—not with focusing

There clearly is a problem in cerebral organization. The corpus callosum controls all those eye motions that have been found to be faulty in dyslexia, especially horizontal tracking, smooth convergence and stable ocular dominance. Fast, accurate interhemispheric "chit-chat" is needed for smooth operation of the eyeballs.

Dyslexia, then, can be succinctly defined as **sub-standard reading in an intelligent person, caused by a transfer delay in the corpus callosum.** This definition has the advantage of distinguishing dyslexia from ADD and ADHD. Unfortunately few professionals know enough to tell the difference, with the result that thousands and thousands of kids today are drugged with medicines like Ritalin. The best a drug can do is tone down the little spitball throwers and make the teacher's life easier.

The definition also explains why dyslectics haven't learned to read in the first place. For a standard reader, you merely pour some phonics into his head when he is young and if you put English phonics into him and he has an English speaking vocabulary, out comes English reading. If he gets French phonics on top of a French vocabulary, out comes French reading. With a dyslectic person, you can put into his brain as much phonics as you want, but it is not going into the side where the software is there to turn it into reading. No matter how hard the teacher or the student tries, the material goes in the wrong place and comes out scrambled.

This explains why remedial reading and other standard teaching approaches don't work well on dyslectic students. You may know your phonics cold and still read "but" for "tub" if you don't keep sequences straight, and if you don't respect punctuation you can still turn into a cannibal, and without understanding the subtleties of grammar and syntax, you won't comprehend what you read, and if you don't use an auditory loop, you can't read unfamiliar words. From the teacher's point of view there is only one thing to do: bypass that sticky corpus callosum, *link those neurons* and get that left brain working.

MERRY CHRISTMAS!

By the time Christmas came that first year when I was using the I CARD and the tapes, it was obvious that something funny was going on. I'd have sworn my boys were actually *reading*. By the end of the year, these intelligent kids, who had taken seven years, most of it in SPED, to achieve a three year gain in reading, clocked in with another three year's gain in only one!

I was ecstatic. I rushed into the office of the SPED director and got the first of a life-long series of put-downs. "Either you fudged the scores or you don't know how to give the tests," he said. He should have fired me, but he didn't, probably because the parents were no longer bugging him. Fortunately for me not everybody was so suspicious. Still, *"The Journal of Learning Disabilities"* probably startled a lot of people when they published an account of the program in 1977. In those days, kids "with special needs" were not required to be in regular classes, so that year I also taught them math, social studies and science, and the faculty complaints disappeared as well. And for the next three years, I kept my job and had the time of my life. Without regular classes, without regular textbooks with facts to memorize and memorize and memorize, I could do what I liked. And without the stress and embarrassment of marks and testing, the kids could enjoy learning. And they did.

Teaching English was a piece of cake. I just supplemented my RfS reading program by reading aloud to them whatever book their classmates were assigned, so they would hear some good literature and could join a conversation with their pals. And of course, I added my own favorites. The kids really ate up "To Kill a Mockingbird" and "The Miracle Worker."

Science was even more fun. The school (why I'll never know) owned a real skeleton, and one time I borrowed it and laid it out on two desks put together. We observed finger bones, ribs, elbows, the curvy spine, knee and hip joints and saw why legs and arms will only bend one way. I had as much fun as the kids did.

In those days you could go into a butcher shop and get a fresh beef heart with one lung attached. (The lung was for cat food, one butcher told me). I brought one in so the kids could see the auricles, the ventricles and the valves and understand the flow from one chamber to another. I gave each student a straw so he could put the end of it into the tube that went to the lung, blow into it and watch the spongy stuff puff up! (It made me think that comparing the hideously diseased real lung of a smoker with a nice healthy real one from a cow would be an excellent part of an anti-smoking campaign). Back in the seventies the National Geographic was selling a globe that showed how the earth would look without water. What a treasure! We looked at deep sea trenches, saw continents diving under each other and causing earthquakes. We saw continental shelves, islands rising from the sea floor, and the obvious match between the shape of South America and Africa. There's no end to the things you can do with a globe like that. We even got into westerlies and the Coriolanos effect.

No wonder I had a ball. Because the kids were not in regular classes, they didn't have to pass multiple choice tests on the contents of a textbook, so while I put them through my reading program two at a time, that left time when I could teach math or tell them stories about everything that fascinated me. And since science is basically finding out how things work—anything, not just what is in a seventh grade science textbook—my conscience was perfectly clear! During those first few years I achieved my two main goals: get a student's reading up to grade level, and let him experience what Richard Feynman has called "The Pleasure of Finding

Things Out." Fortunately, by the time I had gotten their reading levels up to where they belonged, they were also able to take on the next grade without any trouble.

There was only one administrative detail that needed some adjusting, and that was report cards. Because the kids were in SPED they didn't get a mark in a regular subject. This upset our principal who ran the place like the army with strict adherence to rules. I had to point out to him (nicely) that if a child coming into seventh grade with a reading level of third grade, and left at the end of one year with a reading level of sixth grade, he had quadrupled his learning speed! You could hardly give him an F in reading. On the other hand, he would be going into 8th grade two years behind. Couldn't give him an A, either. So I evolved one final report card that had only one letter grade. That grade was for BEHAVIOR, and I told the kids *it had better be an A+*. Then I wrote a short note to the parents explaining what their child's reading level had reached, what we were doing in class in regular subjects and what I had planned for him the following year. Of course you can only do that with six or seven kids. A tutor has it all over a classroom teacher.

During those years many of the experts in the field were still insisting that there was no such thing as dyslexia, or that if the left hemisphere were not being used it must be damaged and therefore could not be changed, or that the results, not being achieved by anyone who *was* anyone in the field, were suspect, or—and this was the best—I was such a wonderful, absolutely delightful teacher that the kids couldn't help but learn! I would have happily agreed with that one if it weren't for the fact that when a few other teachers here and there began using the program, a few of them weren't delightful at all, but their kids learned to read just as well. Added to this nonsense was the undeniable fact that the program was written, taught, and before-and-after tested by the same person and there was no brain scan for validation. That's not science.

But then, neither is phonics, as some teaching programs claim. Writing is an *invention*, arguably the most brilliant idea ever to come from the mind of man. Choosing a written squiggle to represent a language sound and lining the squiggles up in the right order was invented before Hammurabi. If only sound-symbol matching were enough, there wouldn't be any dyslectic people. Clearly something extra is needed from science to explain why a dyslectic brain cannot seem to perform that sound-symbol match when everybody else's brain can. So far it looked as though the CC were the worm in the apple since the kids *could* read without it but could not read if they were using it. But what was the matter with the thing?

In those days a teacher couldn't peek into a student's head and find that his corpus callosum is out of shape. If the child is clearly bright and normal in other ways, how can she figure out why his reading and spelling are so bad? Only a scientist can peek, and they weren't doing it yet.

But maybe you don't have to peek. Dr. Condon, of the high speed photography, had found a delay in transfer time for the whole body, not just the eyes. This implied a problem in some central processing area of the brain. The CC was the only candidate for the job. Another piece of evidence came inadvertantly from a company that made something called an Ober Visagraph which was an eye movement recorder system. They had a device that would record eye motions while a person was reading. This was just what was needed to demonstrate the difference between the eyeball motions of a normal reader and those of a dyslectic reader. The eyes of a dyslectic reader will move to the next word but flick back to the previous one before going on. The eyes of a normal reader move smoothly to the right as they take in one word then move to the next one. But not my boys' eyes! Back went the eyes after each word to the previous one before jumping forward again. Back and forth. Back and forth. This jerky movement can also be seen when a dyslectic person's eyes converge when he is looking at a pencil coming slowly toward his face. The normal person's eyes converge smoothly. The dyslectic one's eyes move in stair-steps, first one, then the other, then the first.

The question still remained as to whether the problem was simply mechanical, involving a poorly constructed CC or whether the brain didn't understand the first word fast enough for it to go on to the next one. Or maybe the eye saw too much area around the word to pick it out quickly. An ingenious scientist named George Pavlidis decided to find out.

Instead of putting a word on the screen, he put a *dot* on, followed by another to the right and so on across the screen. The person had to look at each dot as it appeared, his eyes moving to the right as if reading. The eyes of normal readers moved smoothly across as they looked at the dots. But the eyes of the dyslectic readers? They *still* jumped back and forth! But there was no reading, no comprehension, no word length involved. Just one dot of light.

By now MRI's are in regular use—yes even to study dyslexia!—and the evidence against a malfunctioning corpus callosum has gotten so strong that researchers are finally taking a closer look at it. And the CC is coming out guilty as charged. Today's journals are now full of articles coming right out and saying that an out-of-shape corpus callosum causes dyslexia. My favorite article will always be the one by the Norwegian scientists with the pictures of their funny looking CC's. When they peeked inside, they hit the jackpot. And one of my two favorite scientists will always be Dr. Condon, the psychiatrist with the high-speed camera, who discovered that in a dyslectic individual, the the whole body is out-of-sync with itself, showing that the problem was a mechanical one which showed up everywhere, not just in language handling. And he even measured the time delay with nothing fancier than a high-speed camera! Another favorite scientist is Dr. Pavlidis, who took language out of the equation entirely with his use of dots. But my favorite of all must be Dr. Michael Gazzaniga, with his "one final cognitive path."

NUMBERS, PLEASE

On one memorable September morning in 1998, the principal of a high school told me she would be glad to provide a tutor for one of her pupils who had been diagnosed as dyslectic. I couldn't believe it. Most of the time I would be coldly informed that public schools do not supply tutors for dyslectic kids. They already have all those extra programs, resource rooms, inclusion models, etc, that are taking care of the problem. I was anxious to reduce the cost of tutoring for this nice principal and suggested that she get another dyslectic student and teach them both at once, since the material she would be using was designed to be used with two kids at a time. She answered that, yes, she felt sure they could find another dyslectic student and thought it was a good idea.

How many students were in her school? Two thousand! After taking a deep breath, I told her since 10% of her population were dyslectic, undoubtedly she could locate another one. She stared at me in disbelief. Poor soul.

Like 99.99% of the population, she had no idea there were so many. It is the invisibility factor again.

Estimates by the experts vary from 5% to 20% so 10% is probably close enough. In America years ago, poor reading in general was not due to dyslexia. It was mainly the result of that teaching method popular for decades, which put the United States near the bottom of the heap when people did worldwide tests of reading, math and science. That's why, with the exception of a few super speed-readers of the world, many middle-aged Americans are still iffy readers, and worse spellers. It is a residue of "Whole Language" that was popular in the fifties, sixties and even into the seventies, which eschewed phonics as too boring for their pupils' little brains and taught them to read by recognizing the pattern of each word. This, of course, trained them to use the *right* hemisphere by mistake, practically trying to make them dyslectic! It was only after phonics made a comeback and the dyslectics *still* couldn't read, that you could find out how many there really were.

The other thing that was a fatal mistake in the forties was to abandon teaching spelling rules. Some dingbat once decided that, in his opinion, most of English was irregular, anyhow, so there was no point in teaching spelling rules. And because this misguided theory fit nicely with "Whole Language," people actually believed it. Finally some more intelligent soul actually did a real count instead of guessing and came up with the information that, while 15% of English words are irregular, 85% are either "regular" or "consistent." By consistent, he meant that a certain spelling, like, say,—tion, might not be "regular" but it ALWAYS spelled the sound /shun/ so it only has to be learned once. Over the years I have found, somewhat to my surprise, that whether your lessons include a lot of connected reading or not, if you jam enough spelling rules into your pupil's left angular gyrus, *he learns to read faster*. He even spells somewhat better, but the big improvement is in smooth, connected reading!

Putting aside the results of years of misteaching, we still have enormous numbers of poor readers with miswired brains. In America alone there are over 46,000,000 children in school, of whom more than 5,500,000 are already in Special Education. Two thirds of these SPED kids are there because they are having reading problems, with the other third consisting mostly of children who are retarded, fire-setters, multiply handicapped, or suffering from some medical problem like schizophrenia, clinical depression, or paranoia. That means that there are roughly three and a half million kids just in the US who are dyslexic. And that is just kids. You can further boggle your mind by adding unrecognized adult dyslectics. Now if you take ten percent of the

English-speaking people in the rest of the world—India, Canada, South Africa, New Zealand and Australia, we are up to about 20,000,000 people! And these figures will never go down as long as people continue to have babies. The supply of dyslectic kids will always be about 10% and the demand is not a matter of taste. Dyslexia is very democratic. It bothers all kinds of people equally, showing no preference for race, gender, age (it is never outgrown), ethnicity, or upbringing.

Well, the moral of that story is that there are a lot more dyslectic people in this world than will ever be taught to read, and not just because they will never be identified. The cost would be staggering. Right? Well, yes and no. It would be, if you just look at the way people pay today for special reading lessons. As of this writing, in my school district we have 1162 children on the SPED roles with IEP's (Individual Educational Plan's.) Nearly 1100 of those are dyslectic. We have a couple of hundred teachers and paraprofessionals for this group, at a cost of five and a half million dollars. And that doesn't even include School Psychologists, School Adjustment Counselors, SPED caseworkers, attendance paras, and supplies.

But it gets worse. The unvarnished truth is that all those SPED teachers *don't teach their dyslectic students to read at anywhere grade level no matter how much you spend.* So after blowing all that tax money, we still have

56

kids graduating from high school with reading levels of fifth grade after years of being in SPED.

And that brings up another sore subject. Dropouts. Your true dropout rate is a measure of how many of your *ninth* graders don't go on to graduate from high school. In many schools, something like 30 percent don't finish. That's pretty much the same crowd that couldn't read. Students who are good readers very rarely drop out before getting that diploma. But you don't have to wait until ninth grade to find them. The dyslectic readers are easily identified by sixth grade by comparing their grade-level of reading with their IQ's. Bright kids who can't read are almost invariably dyslexic. Until they are 16, they can only keep on suffering in school because they are not allowed by law to quit. Understandably, many of them figure that if they have the brains of an earthworm, when they turn 16 they will leave school as quickly as possible and get into some sort of job that doesn't humiliate them eight hours a day. But a simple test to find a mismatch between ability and achievement years earlier could catch them before it is too late.

Does this neglect cost the taxpayers money? Oh yes, and not just SPED money. The social costs of dyslexia are extremely high but the payment for wasted talent, jail terms, underutilized intelligence and welfare assistance all come out of somebody else's budget—not that of the school board. The high cost to society of things like depression and underutilized intelligence are impossible to assess. It is the invisibility factor again. So the moderate cases in school remain unidentified while the severe cases are put into an "inclusion" model. This means that the kid has a baby-sitter (read that, aide) who follows him around all day, explains what the teacher means, corrects his spelling and writes down his homework assignments. *But she doesn't teach him to read.*

In high school, the "teaching" consists mostly of homework help and coping skills, such as memorizing the answers in the <u>Driver's Manual</u>. At that level, most teachers will have long since given up the idea that students even *can* be taught to read at their grade level. The lucky kids are given taped textbooks, untimed oral tests, and training on a word processor. Their mothers read everything to them. In spite of all that, they go through life scarred by twelve years of ego-bashing failure, employed at jobs for which they are intellectually over-qualified, depressed, frustrated and exhausted from the constant struggle to maintain their self-respect in a world that is crawling with words they can't handle.

The unlucky ones? They usually drop out after ninth grade. Incidentally, the great majority of male juvenile offenders in local lockups are extremely poor readers and the Orton Society and other investigators have found large numbers of dyslectics among them. They are put in jail and returned to society sometime later with their reading just as bad as ever. The sheriff knows them well. They keep coming back.

The situation is similar to treating pneumonia before the discovery of penicillin. TLC was nice, but it didn't attack the germs that were causing the problem. Once something was found that actually eliminated the germs, the patient could recover quickly. However, you won't cure pneumonia by rubbing penicillin on your arm a couple of times a week. The cure must be put in the appropriate place with the proper timing. In dyslexia the "germ" is a misshapened corpus callosum. So why are schools so reluctant to face dyslexia? Because as far as I know, the only way to achieve grade-level or better reading is to give kids reading lessons no more than two at a time for 45 minutes a day for a year or so while you isolate the lessons to the left side. Say "two-at-a-time" to a school department and watch 'em stare at you. Don't you know that school budgets are already shrinking until they are wrinkled? Way too expensive.

But is it? One SPED teacher can teach 12 kids a day in elementary school for a year, by-passing the CC, wiring the auditory and visual signals together, and have them reading at—sometimes above—grade level. Then they are finished. *After that, they don't need any further intervention*. If the teacher is paid $48,000 a year, that comes to $4000 extra per kid. That's all. No SPED for years and years. No MCAS special tutoring, no School Adjustment Counselors, no attendance Para's, no teachers wasting time on IEP meetings and endless paper work.

In a 2009 study on dropouts done by WBUR and WGBY in Boston, a Northeastern University economics professor, Andrew Sum, found that a high school dropout is eight times more likely than a high school graduate to end up behind bars. And the cost of keeping a person in jail is a mind-numbing $80,000 a year.

The cost of teaching a dyslectic child to read well is about $4800. As our perceptive sheriff always says, pay now or pay later. But why pay at all if closing the science-education gap can save all that money?

THE STUDENTS

The series of kids I had those first happy years of teaching were normal kids with the usual problems that go with adolescence as well as a few of the accidents and tragedies that befall people just because they are alive. If a teacher is going to be breaking the rules as merrily as I was, it is imperative that she become expert at two things: she must know when to change the subject in a hurry and she must know when to turn a blind eye. Sometimes both at once. One morning a bedraggled little boy arrived with brand new sneakers on. Tommy was one of five children of a single, overwhelmed welfare mom. His shoes had been getting worse and worse until the soles began to flop. When he arrived one day wearing a new pair I said something nice about them. He looked pleased and said, "Yeah, I like 'em. My sister stole 'em for me."

"I—, uh, er,—lets get started," I said hastily. The next day I checked with a ten-cent store clerk to see how common the practice was. This was back in the days before the five-and-dime stores had wised up and put their merchandise under glass. "That's right," she said. They come here, look around, find what they need, the kids slide out of their shoes when nobody is looking, Momma hides them under the pile of new ones, puts the new pair on the child and out they go."

A couple of weeks later, Tommy came in proudly wearing a nice new shirt instead of his worn-out one. Mrs. Chicken couldn't bring herself to compliment him on how nice he looked. I still wish I had.

Another boy named Dave made me swallow twice before deciding what to say. It was years ago when I was working in a junior high school and going back and forth to the guidance office to make up my teaching schedule for the fall. I noticed a kid who was sitting in the hall day after day, just sitting. So I stopped, smiled at him and remarked that they were going to charge him rent if he stayed there much longer. He grinned and said that they were trying to put him in the retarded class and he wouldn't go. He didn't sound retarded to me, so with my antenna waving in the breeze, I asked him which was his right hand. He leaned over, pulled up the cuff of his trouser, took a quick look and held up his right hand!

"Wow," I said. "What did you do, have it tatooed someplace?" He giggled and said no, that he had a scar on his right ankle so he could always tell.

Naturally I smelled dyslexia (left-right confusion?) and got him into my class. He was my devoted slave after this dramatic rescue and a bright and hard-working student. But one day he came in and fidgeted and twisted and squirmed and obviously couldn't concentrate. I asked him what was the matter. He told me he needed a nicotine fix, and could he please go to the boy's room?

So then what do you say?

Well, I couldn't teach him the way he was, so I swallowed said that yes, he could **go to the bathroom.** One minute later he came back, sat down quietly and started on his work again.

"Well, that was the fastest cigarette I ever heard of," I couldn't help remarking.

"Oh, I didn't smoke a whole one. There was another kid there who was smoking, so I just took a drag off his and now I'm fine."

This 13 year old lived alone in serious poverty with his largely disabled father. His mom had apparently died a couple of years previously. The boy took care of his dad and did most of the housework. I couldn't help noticing that the considerable clutter in the tiny house included a lot of books which the father read to the boy. Apparently the man had been rather an American history buff, which accounted for the fact that the kid knew all kinds of stuff about this country that had constantly surprised me before I made that home vist. The two nicest things in this boy's life were the soothing feel of a cigarette and being read to by his father.

I think of Dave every time a see one of those oboxious ads by tobacco companies touting their financial support of ballets and *their campaigns to help kids stop smoking!* Hypocrisy inspires the most unladylike language in me so I will only add that Dave deserved a better anodyne than a cigarette.

The saddest unanswerable question in all my years of teaching came from one hapless youngster who must have been one of the unluckiest people alive. His beloved grandmother was fatally ill in the hospital, and it happened that at the moment she died, Tommy was the only person in the room to see her go. A few months later, his father, too, died in the hospital, and again, Tommy happened to be the only person in the room to watch him die. At his father's funeral I found out that his mother was also deathly ill! One week after the father died, the mother died in the hospital and, yes, Tommy had to watch her die, once more, all by himself.

The relatives closed up the house he had lived in and he was moved in with an aunt across the street. They had locked the house, but this child knew a way to jimmy a window and get in. A few days after the third funeral, he came to class and asked if he could ask me something. Apparently he would climb in the window after he got home from school, stand in the doorway of his mother's bedroom from which he could "see" her in her bed and talk with her. His aunt told him he was going crazy, and he asked whether I thought so, too. I assured him that he was certainly not going crazy, but that his brain had suffered from three severe shocks in a row and it was only trying to heal by doing what brains do—visualize something it wanted badly. (I fervently hope to this day that the answer was correct.)

But then came the really unanswerable one. Should he keep on going in and talking to her or stop? What on earth could I tell him? After a long, deep breath I said I thought he ought to do whatever made him feel better and talk to her if it helped. When he didn't need to any more, he would know, and then he could stop. He came to class a couple of days later and told me that he had decided he didn't need to go in any more. Shortly after that, he was sent to live with relatives somewhere in the south. I prayed they were awfully nice people.

Sometimes it works the other way. The kids will come through and make you look good. We operated one year in a little room off the stage in the auditorium which had a solid door with no glass so that you couldn't see who was coming in. The boys were relaxed in their chairs with their feet up on the chair in front while we chatted about some wonderful pictures I had from Life Magazine on ancient Greece. Without warning the door opened and in walked the principal! There was a thud as twelve feet hit the ground at once and a slight scraping of chairs as they all sat bolt upright. And you would have thought that there were six Little Lord Flauntleroys in class. Hands were raised politely, I was Mrs. van den Honert, sensible questions were asked, nobody interrupted anybody. When the door closed behind him, the feet went back up and a comfortable disorder was restored.

"That was pretty good, wasn't it, Mrs. V?" they asked.

"Oh man, you were *wonderful*," I said. In fact it was such an impressive performance that a week later the principal gave us a bunch of big maps of the Mediterranean without my even asking.

It ia pretty hard to teach without learnng something yourself from your students, and one boy I shall call Ray inadvertantly helped me answer a question I am often asked by both teachers and parents. If you transfer language handling out of the artistic right hemisphere, will you upset the balance and decrease artistic or spatial ability? Many of my kids were real artists. I had never seen them lose their drawing ability when they learned to read well. But that was mere speculation because I didn't *want* to believe that I was making them less creative!

Ray was put in my class for math help. He was reading, in the ninth grade, at about a high seventh-grade level. Nobody thought that was too bad, even though, with an IQ of 120, he should have been reading (and spelling) much better than that. His math, however, was dismal. He couldn't add, subtract, multiply or divide. I tested Ray and found a moderate case of dyslexia plus something I had never seen before. I drew a pentagon:

and asked him to copy it. His pentagon looked like this:

Well, I scratched my head and asked him whether he was finished, and he said he thought so, although his didn't really look <u>exactly</u> like mine. Next I drew a Necker cube—one of those glass cubes that every kid draws by making two squares and then connecting the corners:

Ray watched me do it but couldn't duplicate it to save his life! I also found out that he was permanently excused from gym because if you threw a ball to him, he couldn't tell accurately where it was coming from, and he often got hit. (He hated gym with a passion, so that was no problem.) I wrote on his report that I suspected some right-hemisphere damage, and a neurologist who had examined him concurred.

It was obvious from the beginning that Ray was never going to learn arithmetic from any strategies I knew of, so I got permission from the district math coordinator to teach him how to use a calculator. (This was back in the seventies, when such ideas were pretty radical.) It didn't take long to show him how to punch in a numerical problem, but of course he had no idea what to do with a word problem in which he had to decide which function to use. Since his reading clearly needed improving, I decided to abandon the math lessons for awhile. I put him on the earphones and the I CARD and started him on the RfS program instead.

Sometime in April, after his reading had improved dramatically to well above grade level, I began to have a guilty conscience about his math, so I got out the calculator again. After several lessons, I had the feeling that Ray was actually understanding the concepts behind the operations. After six weeks of work this boy could go through a five-step salesman's commission problem (with the calculator, of course) and get a right answer! One day, just out of curiosity, I drew a pentagon and asked him to copy it. He made a nice, closed figure! With my heart in my mouth, I drew a Necker cube and asked him to copy that, and slowly and carefully, he copied that correctly, too! (I never tried to see whether he could catch a ball for fear he might succeed and blow his gym excuse.)

I was so excited I told his last year's teacher and his this year's teacher and his mother and his father and everybody else I could buttonhole! When last heard from, he was in his second year of college and doing nicely. With the calculator, of course. He still can't add, subtract, multiply, or divide, but he told me one day years later that whenever he doodles, he still draws Necker cubes!

I have since seen many serendipitous increases in math comprehension—not calculating, but understanding concepts—after exposure to EL, and there have been no apparent decreases in artistic ability. It leads me to believe that when the brain is forced to process information more normally, each side will operate better. In any case, one side doesn't seem to improve at the expense of the other. But I'm no neurologist, so I can't prove it.

On one memorable occasion I didn't have a chance to prove it. Years ago I had a big, tough kid that nobody else wanted. He was dyslectic, so when I asked for him, the administration was only too glad to turn him over. He was supposed to be learning math as well as reading with me, so I got a bunch of Cuisenaire rods and dumped them on the desk and let him fool around with them for a few minutes while I did something else with the other student.

When I went back to him he had made a beautiful construction with what looked like four towers in the corners and a "building" in the middle. This was a kid right out of the slums, so I wasn't thinking when I laughed and said, "Wow, that looks just like the Taj Mahal!"

"It **IS** the Taj Mahow," he said indignantly. Somewhat startled, I asked him where he had heard about the Taj Mahal, and he said that his mother had it on a calendar at home and it was the most beautiul building in the world.

So the kid was artistic, and a little investigating on my part turned up the information that he had a beautiful singing voice. Well, I figured I knew what to do to tame this one while I got him over his dyslexia and eased his anger at the world. Clearly he needed to take an extra music class, join chorus, and have an art period added to his schedule. While he was excelling in these activities, I would take on his dyslexia so that he wouldn't be embarrassed by bad reading and spelling.

To my surprise, the administration went along with this humane plan. The music teacher was also the director of the chorus but a wild woman who brooked no interference with anything she said. The second day of music class, he was standing up when she came in and he didn't sit down when the rest of the kids did.

"SIT DOWN" she barked at him.

Big mistake.

When he didn't, she marched down the aisle intending to push him down into his seat. But when she got close, he tried to slide his desk forward between them so she couldn't reach him. Unfortunately it didn't just slide: it stuck, tipped over and fell with a thud on the lady's instep, breaking it!

So there went music and chorus. He was transferred to an "alternate" school for bad boys, where there was no music, no art, no chorus, and no special reading program. And certainly no pictures of the Taj Mahow.

SO WHAT IS IT ABOUT MATH?

The oddities in handling words can spill over into the handling of numbers. If he can see *"spin"* and read it *pins* or *nips*, he is not impressed with the order of the letters. A hallmark of dyslexia is left-right confusion. Understandably, a brain that is just as happy to go "owdn" in an elevator after going "pu" is not going to be impressed by the difference between 31 and 13. So there goes the decimal system of notation.

The dyslectic person typically has a deficit in verbal memory which shows up especially in memorizing a series of disconnected facts, like the days of the week or the months of the year. So out the window goes the multiplication table, not to mention the addition facts to twenty.

His verbal sequential memory problem also appears in inability to remember which direction came first if he is given three things to do. Every parent of a dyslectic child knows that if she tells him to do this, then that, and then a third thing, she is wasting her breath. He will have forgotten what the first one was by the time she has finished talking and then can't remember which direction was number two and which number three. If you can't remember what order to do things in, that wipes out long division.

The right hemisphere does not handle abstract grammatical concepts. The difference between, "Take one half *from* seven", and "Take one half *of* seven," is the difference between two prepositions, *of* and *from*. Prepositions are abstract grammatical concepts that the right hemisphere doesn't get, so the problem is totally lost on it. And since word problems in math are largely solved by figuring out what the grammar means in terms of math, you can see why they are mud in the eye of the dyslectic who is using his right hemisphere by mistake. (Word problems are mud in the eye of most kids, dyslectic or not. I don't know why we insist on teaching them. The child who can figure out about the boat going downstream against the current is no more apt to argue reasonably when his little brother "borrows" his Ipod than any other big brother.) There is a general misconception that teaching math makes a person more logical and able to solve life's problems more sensibly than a person who is a mathematical dolt. If you believe that, I have a bridge—. Just read the biographies of a bunch of the world's greatest mathematicians. To put it charitably, they are just as nutty as the rest of us. The reason we teach math is that the world is awash in numbers, and there is no escaping them unless you want to go broke or end up in the clink.

But back to the clueless dyslectic math student. Fractions can be a problem, too. Word-poor dyslectic children don't know what the terms "numerator" and "denominator" really mean, so they don't understand why, if you want to add two fractions, you don't simply add the numerators and add the denominators. Then there was the unconventional approach to fractions that one of my very artistic pupils had. He could draw anything. When he was doing a problem in fractions and he came to an improper one, it looked top-heavy to him, offending his artistic eye. So he would blandly write it other way up and go on with the problem.

Another oddity about dyslectics is an inadequate sense of size—lengths, widths, volumes, money, time, or distances. A dyslectic child will tell you proudly that his Papa makes a thousand dollars a year. I have had a bright junior high school student ask me whether a million is bigger than a thousand and how soon it will be Christmas. A mother will tell her ten-year-old that the school bus will be there in five minutes, but he hasn't a clue as to how long that actually is. What this lack of a feel for quantity has to do with the hemispheres of the brain I haven't the faintest idea, but it is certainly common in dyslexia. And it certainly plays hob with the ability to tell whether an answer is sensible or not, or how good an estimate is. People seldom appreciate how necessary it is to be able to estimate quickly. But estimating is by far what people do the most with math. How many yards of these goods do I need for eight place mats? How much gas to get to Squeedunk? Will I have enough time (or money, these days)?

This lack of a feeling for size prevents a dyslectic child from understanding the place value system. A bright little seventh grade girl I was tutoring said one day that she was in trouble with math and could I help her? (Me? An aged, happy old math major? I couldn't wait). I wrote a number one on the paper and asked her how much it stood for. One. Right. Then I erased it and rewrote it to the left one place, leaving a dash where it had been. How much did it stand for now?

"Uh, . . . two?" she ventured.

By the time I finished, she knew that moving her Number One seven places to the left (towards her) got her all the way to the sun, and if she moved it toward me, in three moves its size was invisible. I often wonder how much early math teachers dramatize the cleverness of the decimal system that can write such huge differences in such small spaces.

Things don't improve much in algebra. A person who will happily read right past the period at the end of a sentence because he doesn't realize that the author has finished stating a fact, is not going to find it easy to understand that

$$2x + y = 5$$

is a sentence that states a fact. And if the order of procedure—you have to do this first before you can do that—throws him, so will long division, not to say algebra.

Incidently, when you explain something rather basic to an adult, you can't be cute about it as you might with a kid. Raising a fraction to higher terms? Tell a kid to put a disguise on it. Reduce it to lower terms? Take the disguise off. It's the same inside. With an adult, you tell him that *when you are teaching a kid,* you compare fractions with costumes because he gets it better that way. Or you can say, "I used to tell my kids that . . . . It's funny how just that one twist helped it make sense to them. Or, "A friend of mine told me that when she was little, she always thought of the . . . . as a . . . . I think that's neat, don't you?"

So stimulating the left hemisphere of the brain helps with math as well as reading. It even might help him understand why he needs to pay off his plastic every month. If you can teach him to read AND pay off his credit card—LOOK OUT WORLD! That one's gonna make it!

GROWNUPS

So far we have only dealt with children with a sticky corpus callosum, but obviously the world is flooded with adults in the same boat. Is it possible to teach an adult the same way—by by-passing the CC and stimulating the left hemisphere? Does it work if you are in your forties? Fifties? It works if you are in your forties. I'm not sure about the fifties for two reasons. I haven't tried it on anyone over 45, and I suspect that by the time you are over that, you have developed all kinds of strategies to keep out of trouble and may not be motivated to take on something out-of-the-box like this program. On the other hand, the human brain is amazingly plastic. You make millions of new connections of dendrites every time you open your eyes, and plenty of elderly people have learned a foreign language.

Dyslectic adults can be found in community colleges, state teachers' colleges, and even occasionally in a state or private university. When they get into academic trouble (usually quite promptly), they may be offered a standard peer tutoring program, but that will not solve the reading problem. Proper screening needs only to be the Tactile Localization test and a writing sample. If the student is smart enough to get into college with dyslexia, you don't have to worry about his IQ. The *specialized* tutoring which will by-pass the corpus callosum can turn college from an exhausting, frustrating and nerve-wracking chore into a reasonable experience. A peer tutoring program that actually fixed the timing problem would be an enormous help because it would enable the student to learn to read properly, not just get outside help with his homework.

But what about the average Joe who will not go to college and is still hampered by his inability to read on his job? Shortly after I devised the RfS program for junior high school children, two women who got interested in it wondered whether the technique would work in older people. They got themselves a grant from the Department of Education in Massachusetts and investigated. They formed three groups of students: one using RfS with the equipment that isolated the verbal signal to the left side, one using RfS just as a phonics program without the equipment, and a popular program they referred to as "the Comparison Curriculum," designed for disabled adult readers and already used in a lot of adult education centers. All were in their twenties or thirties.

Scores were recorded as years and months. A score of 7.9 would mean a gain of seven years and nine months. Obviously the average gain would be 1 year of gain in 1 year of teaching. After the first year the Comparison Curriculum students' rate of gain was .6 times the average, which figures, since dyslectic students are known to improve at about half the speed of the normal reader. The gain for the RfS students, however, was 4.6 times the expected rate! The most startling statistic, however, was in the area of comprehension. The RfS students using the equipment gained at 6.5 times the expected rate, and RfS *even without the equipment* improved at 3.6 times the expected rate.

These scores were so discrepant that the teachers decided not to continue the other curriculum, knowing that there was something much faster for these adults. So instead of being a two year program, as I had hoped, it was a one year affair. I would have expected the DOE in Boston to take a look at what their funds had uncovered and do something about it, but they never did. So adults know it will be years in an adult ed center before they can read and spell well. I have only vast admiration for those who persist.

One of the students in the study using RfS with the equipment was later asked to make a presentation at a conference co-sponsored by the Literacy Coalition of Western Massachusetts. This is what he said:

"The only way I can explain what life is like after learning how to read is by comparing it to when I couldn't read. The one thing I can say up front is the main difference is attitude . . . . When I was asked to speak here today about what life is like after learning how to read, I thought to myself this is going to be a snap. My life has changed tremendously, or so I thought. But when I sat down to write some notes, I found that my life hasn't changed so much, but my attitude toward life has changed tremendously. I had a job before, I had bills that had to be paid, children to bring up, just like any reader. I still have these things to do, but they don't seem to take as much effort. They're not so cold and burdensome. Now they are challenging and fun. FUN, a word I had never associated with life before learning to read. Things were fun, but life wasn't, and that's attitude.

Before learning to read, if there was a job I wanted, I might go and apply for it, and if I did, when sitting in the interviewer's office, after I had taken the employment application and snuck down the street, I would whip out my trusty little cheat sheet so I could fill out the application 'in the privacy of my shame,' and take it back, filled out, of course! Then, sitting in the office, I would think am I a good enough actor to sell this person a defective bill of goods?

The key words here are might, cheat, sheet, disguise, and the big one, the most important one to non-readers, SHAME! Your attitude toward everything is distorted. Now in the same situation I am selling a product that is fully operational—worth the investment to the employer. Not just because I can read, write and spell, but because of the attitude that grows out of it.

Learning to read isn't a magic pill that changes your life overnight, but it is a magic pill that lets you stand just tall enough to be eye to eye with others. To the non-reader who wonders if the effort to learn is worth it is this: there is no pot of gold at the end of the rainbow, but there is a rainbow. And to those of you who wonder if teaching the learning-disabled is worth it, Yes, and thank you."

But then there was Al. He was a seventh grade student in my first year of teaching, and although he went from a second grade level to about fourth it was some help, but when he went into eighth grade and subsequently dropped out he was essentially illiterate. He took up carpentry, worked with his father for awhile, got married, fathered a child, couldn't make a living, fought with his father, took up drinking, became an alcoholic and spent a few weekends in the local lockup for fighting, loudly blaming all his problems on dyslexia. Several years later, he turned up on my doorstep, dried out and repentant, still with a wife and kid to support, and asked whether I would start again and teach him to read. This time it went better, and in a few weeks it became apparent that he really was going to succeed! Although his lessons were free, he began skipping more and more frequently, and finally he just stopped coming. Then it hit me. He had used dyslexia as his excuse for all his problems, and when he was about to lose it, he couldn't face life without his prop.

EVERYBODY ELSE

I often watch "Judge Judy" and admire her ability to zero in with sharp questions that extract just the information she needs, whether the hapless plaintiff wants her to or not. But one time I got so mad at her that I actually found her web site and wrote her a note explaining something in VERY CLEAR language—polite, but VERY CLEAR. The plaintiffs were twin high school boys who had some complaint against a boy who had done something wrong to them. I have forgotten the exact circumstances—and the other kid had a countersuit against the twins because they had biffed him good.

Judge Judy ascertained that the twins were poor students at school and the butt of endless jokes, but what she didn't see was the depression and quiet despair in their eyes that marked them as dyslectics. Before the end of the program she delivered a stern lecture to them on working harder at school and getting better grades so that they would not be the victims of teasing.

This was too much for me, so I explained in my e-mail about dyslexia and how kids, in spite of monstrous efforts to learn, were bullied in school—often right under the eyes of their teachers—for something for which they were not responsible etc., etc., etc., implying that she should find out before the show whether dyslexia was a contributing factor in a case.

I never heard from her, of course, and I haven't seen any of her cases since then in which bullying in school was a factor, so I don't know whether she reads her e-mail or not. On the other hand, I have not seen her lecture a kid on working harder in school, either.

It is bad enough when people in the general public make a child's life worse because they don't know anything about the subject, but when a SPED teacher's ignorance makes the kid miserable, I get my knickers in a twist.

I got an e-mail the other day from a mother who was upset because her little boy wanted to take trumpet lessons in school so he could be in the school band. He had been told that because he was dyslectic and couldn't read, he wouldn't be able to read music, either, so he wouldn't be allowed to take trumpet! The mother was extremely upset and I don't blame her. Imagine what it did to that poor child's ego to be put down once more as inadequate, prevented from doing something that would have been really fun, and made, yet again, to look

stupid in the eyes of those lucky pals who were allowed
to play in the band.

Even if the music teacher didn't know anything about
dyslexia, she should have known that reading words
and reading music are totally different processes that
have nothing whatever to do with each other. When
you read music, you are matching some little black
dots to a place on a fence which you must coordinate
with a finger or arm position. It is strictly a spatial
and rhythmic task with no linguistic content. There
are professional musicians who are severely dyslectic,
speed readers who couldn't carry a tune in a paper bag,
speed readers who are excellent musicians, and dyslectic
people who are totally tone deaf. The two conditions
are unrelated.

But when it comes to mind-boggling disregard for the
feelings of children, the top prize does not go to anybody
in the general public. It goes to the Supreme Court of the
United States. Back in 1974 they actually decided that
it is perfectly all right for a lazy or incompetent teacher
to repeatedly humiliate students in order to save herself
some work. The question at hand was the practice of
having students correct each others' tests and/or read out
grades for the whole class to hear. Congress had passed
a law that protected the privacy of student's educational
records "such as a transcript." The Bush administration

and the Supreme Court decided that Congress didn't mean things like classroom tests or teacher's notes. Well, they can't read the minds of the people in Congress, and neither can I. So my guess is as good as theirs. My reading of "educational records" includes anything that a student writes that gets a grade. After all, his grades are what go into his final transcript, and his transcript is nobody's bloody business but his.

Their Eminences had a variety of cute reasons why humiliating a dyslectic student in class is well worth saving a few minutes of teacher time. One of them said, "It is a way to teach material again in a new context, and it helps show students how to assist and respect fellow pupils." (Never mind that the case revolved on the problem that the other students ridiculed the dyslectic student's mistakes and called him a dummy. It is an interesting interpretation of *assist* and *respect*.) Another said, "Correcting a classmate's work can be as much a part of the assignment as taking the test, itself." He didn't explain what was to be gained by having a student see what mistakes other kids made. I thought that analyzing student errors was the teacher's job, not the students'.

With the possible exception of high school English teachers, who sometimes have a teaching load of 125 students, any competent teacher can figure out ways to keep her grading chores to a reasonable level. But the important issue here is not the teacher's work load, but the assmption that it is perfectly OK to deliberately embarrass a child because of something that is not his fault and is beyond his control.

It has been said that the most devastating and long-lasting human emotion is humiliation. To subject a kid to years of it is, in my expert opinion, a particularly cruel form of child abuse, and a teacher who permits it to take place in her classroom should be fired. It is not a coincidence that some of the teen-age, middle-class murderers of our day are dyslectics who have been driven beyond endurance from a lifetime of taunts from their classmates and unfair accusations of laziness, stupidity, and bad attitude from their teachers.

These "justices" appeared to find nothing unjust in forcing a child by law into a situation where he will be subjected for years to psychological abuse. This kind of abuse often has life-long consequences which are just as severe as the result of sexual abuse. Why is one form of humiliation illegal and the other tolerated?

I know why they decided this way. They all got good marks in school. I invited them to take off those black robes, step down from their ivory tower and take a look at the real world. Some of those "dummies" have IQ's that top theirs.

WHEN RIGHT IS RIGHT

If you want to play piano, your fingers will need a lot of exercise until they are fast and strong. But if you try to play a Mozart sonata with only speed and strength, it will sound as though you are R2 D2 banging away. To turn strength and facility into music, you need help from the right hemisphere where emotions and beauty are located. And if you want to read, and all you know is phonics, you may turn into what is called a hyperlexic, or a person who can read like a streak but doesn't comprehend a word he reads. To turn words into ideas, you again need help from the right hemisphere where emotions, beauty, subtlety and context will give you meaning.

It's your right side that says, "Oh WOW!" when you look up from your book and see a spectacular sunset exploding over a lake in Maine. Your right gives you that feeling you get when you look at a little furry puppy, or a Polar bear cub, or even a new-born hippo if its mom is there. Your left side says small hippo. Your right says "It's so cute!" even if it has a face that only a mother could love.

If the left side reads about a kitchen scene when a pot of stew falls on the floor and spills all over the place, its exact words describe the scene—slippery slop on the floor, baby crawling over toward the hot mess, Daddy just coming home, nothing left for dinner. And from those words, the right provides the feelings. But the right side is notorious for not caring about left-right sequencing. If it is doing the reading about the above kitchen scene, and instead of reading POT, it should read TOP—The top fell on the floor—So we need contributions from both sides to turn words into ideas.

Your right likes music, recognizes beauty, thinks puns are funny, sympathizes with others, wants peace in the world. It hates the idea that millions of kids are starving, enjoys the rush of skiing down a steep slope. It recognizes faces, loves to dance, laughs at jokes. It makes us human. It only gets us into trouble when it tries to usurp the specialty of the left side and take over deciphering written language.

The truth is, the world requires many, many varieties of love to make civilization feasible. The left side is clever. The right side is—well, *nice.* Reading isn't the only area where we could use a better balance between the two.

And my s D-i-n mike
Ziac Red
Watyare bib
The Fgr a

Boy 7½ yrs, IQ 105   2nd grade
before training

---

magnet   upset

until   oxen

admit

              sunlit

after 32 lessons with
        EL

7 yr old boy IQ 118

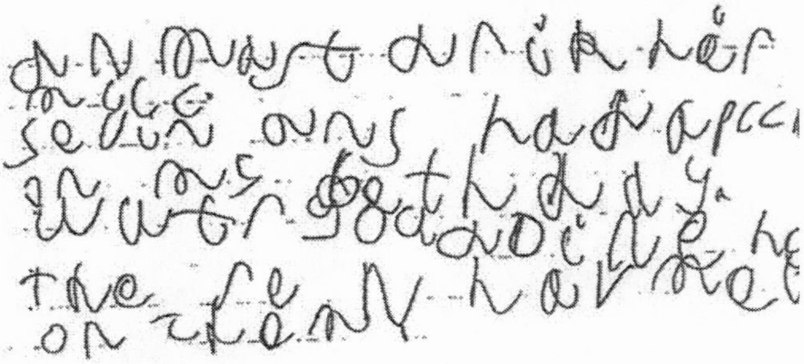

~~After~~ 4 months' training 1/2 1/4

Fish that is not fresh stinks.
I itch to get at my lunch.
You Rush in the clutch.
Had me that crash hellmet

Writing Samples

Boy 7yrs old, second grade

an moSt dran K kern
k ganve antS had a pt
k on my hams tan wa
quit are ydu bo ird hjer
The rosse nrenye buds or
then
Some pople come arve

She kept the Lamp and clock in the
atic.

Dump the clams into the picnic basket.

At dusk the ducks swam in to get
get bugs.

2nd grade age 7, after 4 months' training

30123330R00067

Made in the USA
Lexington, KY
19 February 2014